YOUR KNOWLEDGE HAS VALUE

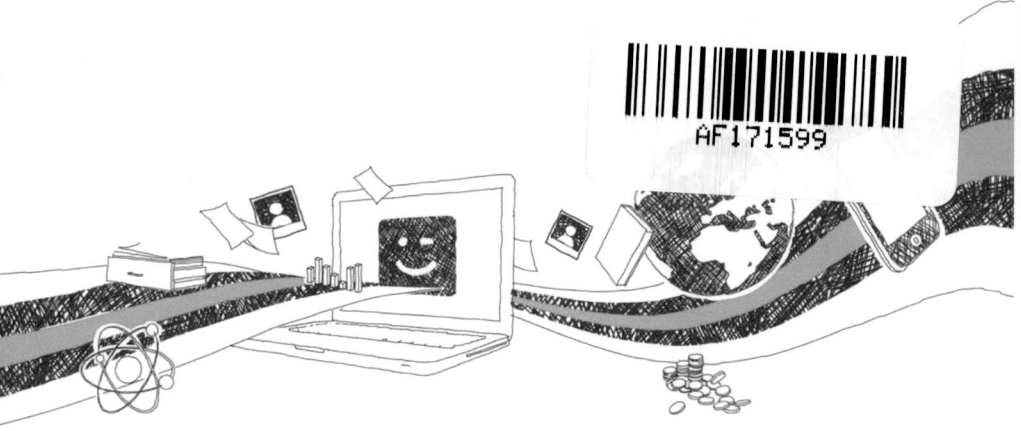

- We will publish your bachelor's and master's thesis, essays and papers

- Your own eBook and book - sold worldwide in all relevant shops

- Earn money with each sale

Upload your text at www.GRIN.com
and publish for free

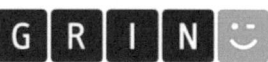

Bibliographic information published by the German National Library:

The German National Library lists this publication in the National Bibliography; detailed bibliographic data are available on the Internet at http://dnb.dnb.de .

This book is copyright material and must not be copied, reproduced, transferred, distributed, leased, licensed or publicly performed or used in any way except as specifically permitted in writing by the publishers, as allowed under the terms and conditions under which it was purchased or as strictly permitted by applicable copyright law. Any unauthorized distribution or use of this text may be a direct infringement of the author s and publisher s rights and those responsible may be liable in law accordingly.

Imprint:

Copyright © 2016 GRIN Verlag, Open Publishing GmbH
Print and binding: Books on Demand GmbH, Norderstedt Germany
ISBN: 9783668351981

This book at GRIN:

http://www.grin.com/en/e-book/344667/cold-chain-management-and-effective-delivery-of-immunization-services

Bruce Wembulua

Cold chain management and effective delivery of immunization services

GRIN Publishing

GRIN - Your knowledge has value

Since its foundation in 1998, GRIN has specialized in publishing academic texts by students, college teachers and other academics as e-book and printed book. The website www.grin.com is an ideal platform for presenting term papers, final papers, scientific essays, dissertations and specialist books.

Visit us on the internet:

http://www.grin.com/

http://www.facebook.com/grincom

http://www.twitter.com/grin_com

The role played by cold chain management in effective delivery of immunization services.

WEMBULUA SHINGA BRUCE

Student of online Advanced Post Graduate Diploma in Tropical Medicine, Surveillance and Immunization – Master of Science in health management

James Lind Institute.

This paper explains the role played by cold chain management in effective delivery of immunization services within a country.

Table of Contents

INTRODUCTION 2

CHAPTER 1. COLD CHAIN TEMPERATURE MONITORING 3

   1. Recommended safe temperature range 3

   2. The Cold-chain Monitor 4

   3. The Vaccine Vial Monitor 4

CHAPTER 2. THE COLD CHAIN SYSTEM LOGISTICS 6

   1. Essential elements of cold chain 6

   2. The Role of Cold Chain and Vaccine Logistics Management 7

REFERENCES 9

INTRODUCTION

In the Greek mythology Aesculapius and Hygieia, two gods of health, have been respectively referred to as therapy and prevention gods. In the twentieth century, Medicine still retains those two concepts as two fundamental ways of maintaining people healthy. Vaccination is a powerful means of prevention ever discovered since it provide the immunity that comes from natural infection without the consequences of natural infection (Plotkin et al. 2011, Offit and Moser, 2011). People are consequently protected from harmful infections before even they come in contact with the disease. Immunoglobulins translated from mothers to their infants confers immunity almost for 3 months after birth for pertussis and 12 months after birth for measles. Since then, vaccination combined with adequate food consumption appear to be "magic bullets "which can improve children's health given their vulnerability (Montgomery 2013, Public Foundation of the Vaccination Research Center 2015)

All vaccines are thermo-sensitive; exposure to extremes of temperature can irreversibly affect their potency and effectiveness. They need subsequently in addition to an appropriate preparation, to be properly stored and distributed (WHO 2016). The success of an immunization program depends on the capacity of the system to continuously maintain the vaccines into recommended temperature range of +2ºC to +8ºC during their transport, storage and distribution. In such an environment, vaccines are protected from both heat and cold. The system that ensures vaccines are transported and stored at and within the recommended temperature range from the place of their manufacture to the point of vaccine administration is called the "cold chain" (New Zealander's Ministry of Health 2012, University of Auckland 2013). The cold chain plays a crucial role to maintain the potency and efficiency of vaccines throughout the immunization process. A network of cold stores, refrigerators, freezers, and cold boxes ensure that vaccines are not exposed to heat or freezing during their transportation, storage, and distribution from factory to the point of use (Sahay, Gupta and Menon 2016; Shendurnikar, and Agrawal 2005).

CHAPTER 1. COLD CHAIN TEMPERATURE MONITORING

Given the vaccine potency is temperature dependent, timely identifying temperature-related events through closer temperature monitoring and measuring devices is vital as it empower health care worker to take meaningful action to reduce the likelihood of product damage.

1. Recommended safe temperature range

It is worthwhile to put a particular emphasis on the fact that the full potency of a vaccine depends on the respect of its safe temperature range. This safe range varies between vaccines and between stages of the cold chain (WHO, 2006). The table below gives the WHO recommended safe temperature ranges of some common vaccines.

Table 1. The WHO-recommended safe temperature ranges (WHO 2006:2).

	Primary vaccine store		Intermediate vaccine store		Health centre	Health post
		Region	District			
OPV	-15°C to -25°C					
BCG						
Measles	WHO no longer recommends that freeze-dried vaccines be stored at -20°C. Storing them at -20°C is not harmful but is unnecessary. Instead, these vaccines should be kept in refrigeration and transported at +2°C to +8°C.					
MMR						
MR						
YF						
Hib freeze-dried						
Meningococcal A&C					All vaccines are recommended to be stored at +2°C to +8°C	
HepB						
IPV						
DT	+2°C to +8°C These vaccines are freeze sensitive and must never be frozen					
DTP						
DTP-HepB						
Hib liquid						
Td						
TT						

2. The Cold-chain Monitor

The cold-chain monitor is of the common instruments used to show exposure to temperature above the safe and recommended range during storage, transportation and distribution processes (NPCS Board of Consultants & Engineers 2015). The Freeze Watch and the DT and TT shipping indicator are also used for the same purpose (WHO, 2006).

The commonly used cold-chain monitor is a thermo-sensitive chemical indicator in a card (e.g. WHO Vaccine Cold-Chain Monitor). It is entirely heat-stable as long as it has not been activated and no colour change must occur, regardless of the temperature to which it was exposed. Once the cold chain monitor is activated, usually by pulling the tag and physically removing trigger strip, it is recommended to place it inside each cold box or vaccine carrier until their final destination is reached. Being thermo-sensitive an activated cold chain monitor gives a different reaction as the temperature varies. For example it turns blue on an exposure to temperature of more than 10°C. At each point of arrival and departure, the card should be checked for any change in color and the information filled in. Finally, it is sent to a predetermined laboratory for careful checking of any weakness in the cold-chain preservation (Vlok 2007, Mc Guire 2015).

3. The Vaccine Vial Monitor

Vaccine vials exposed to unsafe temperature are at high risk of losing their potency. The vaccine vial monitor (VVM) is a special tool allowing registration of effect of heat on individual vials of vaccine. The VVM is a label containing a heat-sensitive material placed on a vaccine vial to register cumulative heat exposure (Parthasarathy 2016:236). It is noticeable by a circle with a small and lighter colored square inside (Fig. 1). Correctly managed the VVM find out about weaknesses in the cold chain ensuring that the vaccines have not been damaged by excessive exposure to heat when they are taken beyond the cold chain to children who have no access to fixed health facilities (Jamison et al. 2006). The inner square of VVM, lighter in color at the starting point, becomes irreversibility darker as the temperature worsens. A direct relationship exists between rate of colour change and temperature: the lower the temperature, the lower the colour change; the higher the temperature, the faster the colour change (Parthasarathy 2016).

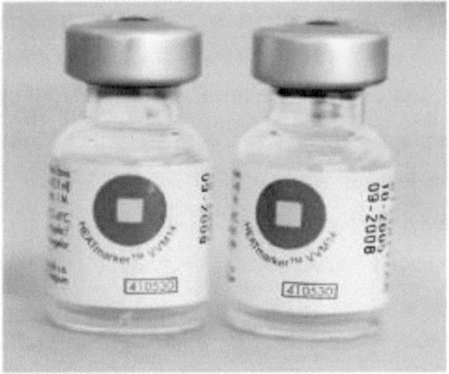

Fig.1. the Vaccine Vial Monitor (Parthasarathy 2016:236).

CHAPITRE 2. THE COLD CHAIN SYSTEM LOGISTICS

1. Essential elements of cold chain

The cold chain must never be broken. To satisfy this principle, the cold chain should not be regarded just as a material problem referring to the storage of vaccines only (Shendurnikar, and Agrawal 2005). Health workers at all levels are often responsible for maintaining a proper continuity of the chain since its integrity is not ensured on the only use of adequate equipment. People handling the vaccine should properly be trained and oriented about what should be undertaken while vaccines are being transported to township and villages, and county levels, or while they are being used during immunization sessions (Sahay, Gupta and Menon 2016; New Zealander's Ministry of Health 2012).

In order to preserve potency and effectiveness of a vaccine up to the point of use a vast well-organized cold chain infrastructure is required. This should have a network of Vaccine Stores, Walk-in-coolers (WIC), Walk-in-freezers (WIF), Deep Freezers (DF), Ice lined Refrigerators (ILR), Refrigerated trucks, Vaccine vans, Cold boxes, Vaccine carriers and icepacks from national level to states up to the outreach sessions (UNICEF 2010). It is important to remind that the simple availability of the best equipment does not ensure vaccine potency unless the staff handling the vaccine have been properly trained and assigned.

Once suitable equipment to store and transport vaccines using adequate transport facilities are timely available to a well-trained staff, the remaining important concern to tackle is the maintenance. Zuckerman and Jong have proposed ten critical elements for a successful maintenance of the cold chain in a travel health clinic as followed:

- Written cold-chain policies and procedures
- All staff responsible
- Designated immunization coordinator
- Vaccine handling requirements
- Cold-chain management equipment and supplies

- Monitoring and documenting vaccine temperature control
- Receiving vaccine supplies
- Vaccine storage and storage troubleshooting
- Vaccine wastage, and
- Transporting vaccines off-site (Zuckerman and Jong 2010).

2. The Role of Cold Chain and Vaccine Logistics Management

Africa dwells larger rates of morbidity and mortality among children as vaccine preventable diseases burden. Proper Immunization campaigns allowing the administration of potent vaccines is one of the most powerful strategies to tackle this issue across all sections of the at-risk population (Samant et al. 2007).

Given immunization against a disease is achieved only if a potent vaccine is administered. Since the introduction of costly vaccines that are sensitive to freezing, the recent tendency has shifted from protecting vaccines just from heat to an overall protection from exposure to cold as well as heat. WHO guidelines for international transport of vaccines have subsequently now include specific recommendations for each category of vaccine, including freeze sensitivity. The next critical level of the vaccine management system concerns national cold stores. These should equally be given importance as failure at that level where vaccines are received, stored, and distributed can also result in results in wastage and unnecessary costs to the national program (Chiodini 2014). The cold chain and vaccine logistics management remains indeed at any level, the backbone, the left and right hands of immunization programs. A poor cold-chain which affects the potency of the vaccine severely may cause vaccine to have no effect on the immunity of the "immunized" person (UNICEF 2010, Vlok 2007).

In many developing countries, conditions are such that it is difficult for the cold chain to be maintained (Kortum 2010). Vaccination programs may need to be performed in remote areas for power is non-existent or power cuts occurs regularly and where road and transport render them difficult to access. Cold chain handlers have the heavy responsibility to improve the immunization coverage of mothers and children by providing safe and potent vaccines and logistics in time (UNICEF 2010, Chiodini 2014). Whenever they suspect that a container of vaccine has not been properly transported or stored, they must throw it rather than risk using inactive vaccine. With the advent of Vaccine Vial Monitors (VVMs) and Freeze watch indicators that provide accurate records of the temperature history though out the storage or transport processes, there have been a significant reduction in vaccine wastage (Kortum 2010). No matter whether vaccines are supplied centrally or purchased directly from the manufacturer as is the case with travel vaccines, the financial burden of wastage should be whenever possible avoided.

To be successful emphasis on optimum protection from correctly stored vaccines is paramount. A clear protocol for ordering, storing and handling vaccines should be available in the workplace to provide detailed information on the roles and responsibilities of all those involved. This will thus reduce the risk of compromising the quality, efficiency and safety of the vaccine, and improving the service for patients (Chiodini 2014). The WHO - UNICEF Effective Cold Store Management Initiative encourages countries to procure equipment and adopt management and training policies that fully protect vaccines both in national and intermediate vaccine stores. At the country level, emphasis is being put on the use of new tools, such as the vaccine vial monitor (Jamison et al. 2006).

REFERENCES

1. Vlok, M. E. (2007). *Manual of Community Nursing and Communicable Diseases: A Textbook for South African Students*. Juta & Co, Ltd.
2. Chiodini, J. (2014). "Safe storage and handling of vaccines". in *Continuing Professional Development*. Nursing Standard/RCN publishing 28 (25): 42-45.
3. Jamison D.T. et al. (2006). *Disease Control Priorities in Developing Countries*. 2d ed. New York. Oxford University Press.
4. Kortum R. R. (2010). *Biomedical Engineering for Global Health*. Cambridge university press.
5. Mc Guire, G. (2015). *Handbook of Humanitarian Health Care Logistics: Designing the Supply Network and managing the flows of information and health care Goods in humanitarian assistance during complex political emergencies in low-resource settings.* 3d ed. [online] available from http://www.humanita rianhealthcarelogistic.com [26-11- 2016].
6. Ministry of Health (New Zealand) (2012). *National Guidelines for Vaccine Storage and Distribution*. Wellington: Ministry of Health.
7. Montgomery, H. (2013) *Local childhoods, global issues*. 2d ed. Bristol, the Policy Press.
8. NPCS Board of Consultants & Engineers (2015). *The Complete Book on Cold Storage, Cold Chain & Warehouse (with Controlled Atmosphere Storage & Rural Godowns.* New Delhi, NIIR project consultancy Services.
9. Offit, P.A., Moser, C.A. (2011). *Vaccines & Your Child: Separating Fact from Fiction*. New York, Columbia University Press.
10. Parthasarathy, A. (2016). *IAP Textbook of Pediatrics*. 6th ed. New Delhi, Jaypee Brothers Medical Publishers (P) Ltd.
11. Plotkin, S.A., Walter, A., Orenstein, A., Offit, P.A. (2011). *Vaccines*. 5th ed. Saunders Elsevier.
12. Public Foundation of the Vaccination Research Center (2015). *Vaccination and children's health*. [Online] available from http://www.yoboseshu-rc.com/ [26-11-2016].

13. Sahay, B.S., Gupta, S.V., and Menon, C. (2016). *Managing Humanitarian Logistics*. New-York. Springer.
14. Samant Y. et al. (2007). "Evaluation of the cold-chain for Oral Polio Vaccine in a Rural District of India". in *Public Health Reports*. 122(1):112-121.
15. Shendurnikar, N. and Agrawal, M. (2005). *Immunization for children*. 2[d] ed. Hyderabad, India. Paras Medical Publisher.
16. UNICEF, Department of Health & Family Welfare Ministry of Health and Family Welfare Government of India (2010). *Handbook for Vaccine & Cold Chain Handlers*. Available from ‹ http://www.nccvmtc.org/PDF2/2_070. pdf.› [28-6- 2016].
17. University of Auckland: Immunization advisory Center (2013). *The essential cold chain: Factsheet for health professionals*. Standards Cold Chain 2013-1210V01 Available from ‹http://www.immune.org.nz/sites/default /files / resources/StandardColdChainImac20131210V01Final.pdf. › [28-6- 2016].
18. WHO, Department of vaccines and other biologicals. (2006). *Temperature sensitivity of vaccines*. Geneva, WHO/IVB/06.10. [Online] available from http://apps.who.int/iris/bitstream/10665/69387/1/WHO_IVB_06.10_eng.pdf [26-11- 2016].
19. WHO, Regional office for Europe (2016). *Vaccine cold-chain management*. Available from ‹http://www.euro.who.int/en/health-topics/disease-pre vention.› [28-6- 2016].
20. Zuckerman J.N., Jong, E. C. (2010). *Travelers' Vaccines*. 2[d] ed. Shelton, People's Medical Publishing House – USA, Ltd (PMPH-USA).

YOUR KNOWLEDGE HAS VALUE

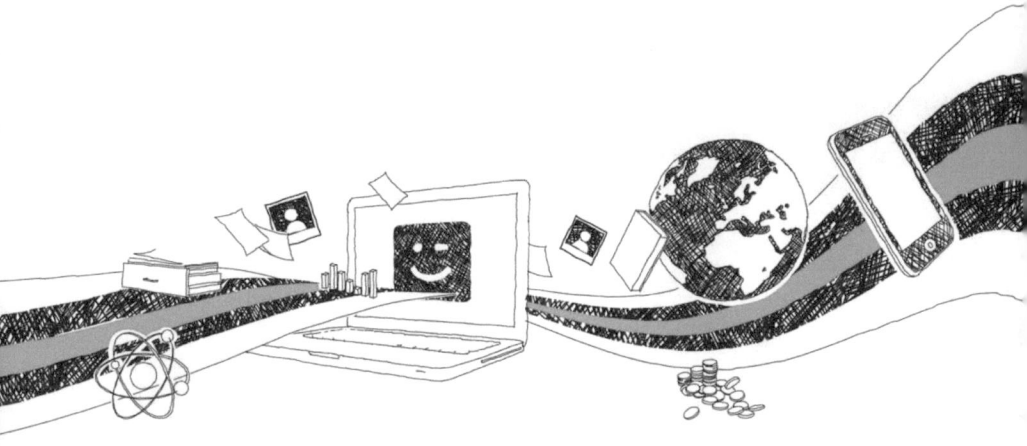

- We will publish your bachelor's and master's thesis, essays and papers

- Your own eBook and book - sold worldwide in all relevant shops

- Earn money with each sale

Upload your text at www.GRIN.com and publish for free

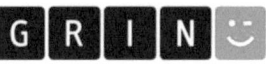